Understanding Hug

Graham R.V. Hughes

Understanding Hughes Syndrome

Case Studies for Patients

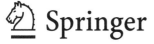 Springer

Graham R.V. Hughes, MD, FRCP
The London Lupus Centre
London Bridge Hospital
London
UK

ISBN: 978-1-84800-932-5   (hardcover)   e-ISBN: 978-1-84800-376-7
ISBN: 978-1-84800-375-0   (softcover)
DOI: 10.1007/978-1-84800-376-7

British Library Cataloguing in Publication Data

Library of Congress Control Number: 2008940862

Printed on acid-free paper

Springer Science + Business Media
springer.com

There are two new diseases of the late 20th century: AIDS and the Antiphospholipid Syndrome

(M. Vilardell, Dean, University of Barcelona)

Foreword

I am honoured, privileged, and grateful that Professor Hughes has allowed me to write a few words at the beginning of his book.

Honoured that he is my professor, my educator, my life support, and my doctor.

Privileged that I can take this opportunity to say a few words. To patients, doctors, families, to "the world at large" as Thomas Crowne would say. To have my thoughts and concerns, my experiences and suggestions, read and maybe even considered is a real privilege indeed!

Grateful to have this opportunity to express my gratitude to my parents, Suzy Bardos-Fischer, and my father, Jacques Mendelson-Fischer. They never gave up, and taught me the same, and because of this, I am still around today to give Professor Hughes such a hard time.

Thousands of people every year find themselves in this similar and strange predicament – suddenly the body starts failing, often no longer able to perform that which it should be able to. Feeling as if we are "falling apart", unusual symptoms, nothing like most doctors have ever seen. We go from doctor to doctor, searching for the answer to the same simple question: "WHY is this happening to me?" Sadly, the answer is rarely found.

Thousands have walked this scary, lonely, confusing road – the same road that I passed not so long ago. I barely made it through this long journey, of 30 or more years, of 30 or more doctors, of 30 or more hospitalizations, of 30 or more mistakes and misdiagnoses. Many times it was a relief when a doctor admitted "I don't know!" rather than the usual diagnosis of hysterical paralysis or that I was crazy.

Then one day, a doctor suggested that I see Professor Hughes in London, England. Off we went, hoping for the best, but fearing that this would be a "31st try!" But when Professor Hughes appeared, he was nothing like I expected, yet everything I had hoped for. Here was this little man, with a big heart and immense knowledge. A "real doctor", the one who actually take the time to listen to a patient. He ran tests, did examinations, and asked questions, surprisingly, always listening attentively to my reply. After some time he said, "I believe I have solved the puzzle!"

Finally, thanks to Professor Hughes, years of searching, years of pain and anguish of not knowing "what was happening?" – was finally over. Diagnosis was made and confirmed by blood tests.

Hughes syndrome with damage to the aortic valve of the heart. Now, we could start on the road to getting better.

On behalf of all the "unwell" people like myself, I thank you and applaud you, Professor Hughes, who after receiving the honor of having your "discovery" named after yourself, you never slowed down, quite the contrary, now you won't stop till you find its cure.

Eternal gratitude forever.

Linda Fischer

Preface

It has been my privilege to have spent a lifetime in medicine, and in particular to have defined a syndrome – an illness – which is not only common but also potentially treatable.

The discovery of "sticky blood" (or more prosaically "The antiphospholipid syndrome" or Hughes syndrome) came out of years of observation of patients with a disease called lupus. I had always been interested in the neurological or "brain" aspects of lupus and spent a number of years studying mechanisms of brain inflammation.

In 1975–1976, I spent a year setting up a rheumatology center and lupus unit in Jamaica. Here, I observed a number of young women with a form of viral paralysis. Interestingly, some of them carried an antibody in their blood directed against "phospholipid" – one of the components of brain and spinal cord.

It quickly became apparent that individuals who had "antiphospholipid antibodies" suffered from a tendency not only to develop brain and spinal cord symptoms but also a tendency to develop both vein and artery thrombosis ("sticky blood").

Crucially, we found that the condition was not confined to patients with lupus, but occurred in others – for example, in patients with migraine, with stroke, with memory loss – and in women with recurrent miscarriage.

We gave the syndrome the name "antiphospholipid syndrome" (APS) – and some years later, my colleagues in the now biannual international APS meeting honored me by naming it the Hughes syndrome.

The joy of the discovery is that it is not only potentially treatable – but, with the simple blood tests available, also allows prediction of future risks and their prevention.

Any illness can be devastating. None more so than a mysterious "new" disease, still not widely taught in medical school. So often, the best lessons come from the patients themselves. That is why, in this short volume, I have selected 50 case histories from patients who have attended my clinic, with the aim of painting a picture of the spectrum that is Hughes syndrome.

This short volume began life as "The Brain and Other Animals," written for patients and distributed by the charity "The Hughes Syndrome Foundation" (www.hughes-syndrome.org). I have made minor changes only, with the aim of keeping the lessons concise and pithy, and, I hope, not too "medical."

I am grateful to Linda Fischer whose enthusiastic and critical support made this publication possible. I am also grateful to Sandy Hampson, Melanie Draper, and Sharminy Ragunathan for advice and help with the manuscript and Victoria Lenzoi Lee for the wonderful illustrations found throughout this volume.

Graham Hughes
The London Lupus Centre
London Bridge Hospital
London SE1 2PR
www.londonlupuscentre.com

Contents

Introduction: "Sticky Blood"

What do the following have in common: headaches, blood clots, memory problems, balance disorders, poor circulation, ... and ... in pregnant women, a tendency to recurrent miscarriage?

The answer is that all can be symptoms of "sticky blood" – a tendency of blood to "sludge" or clot inside blood vessels.

In 1983, we identified a new syndrome. It was distinguished by a tendency to clot both in veins and (very significantly) in arteries and could be easily diagnosed by simple blood tests.

The organs particularly susceptible to "sticky blood" are the brain, and, in pregnancy, the placenta, leading to recurrent pregnancy loss. Such has been the importance of the discovery that the syndrome is now recognized as the commonest treatable cause of recurrent miscarriage.

In 1983, when we described the clinical syndrome, we also set up laboratory assays to detect "anticardiolipin antibodies." This test led us to call the condition "The Anticardiolipin Syndrome." Later, this was changed to "Antiphospholipid Syndrome." Even that title was not totally exact, as, for example, proteins played an important role. So, in 1994, at the eighth international conference on the subject in Louvain, my colleagues proposed the simpler title "Hughes Syndrome."

During the past 25 years, knowledge of the subject has grown, and publications, research meetings, and conferences have recognized the importance of the disease – embracing cardiologists, hematologists, neurologists, surgeons, psychiatrists, obstetricians, GPs, ... , and of course patients.

The very first lesson for all medical students is "listen to the patient, for (s/he) is telling you the diagnosis."

In the case of Hughes syndrome, this guideline is doubly important. Here, the physician is presented with a "new" disease with features as diverse as forgetfulness, fatigue, headache, miscarriage, and blood clots.

Once a year the Hughes Syndrome Foundation runs a patients' forum. This year, Kate Fitzpatrick, manager of the charity, ran a questionnaire among the patients attending the meeting, enquiring about various symptoms such as balance problems, sleep disturbance, and so on. While not particularly "scientific," some of the figures are revealing, highlighting some possibly underrecognized features of the syndrome. I have included some of these "pie-charts" in this volume.

The good news is that despite its clinical complexity, Hughes syndrome/ the antiphospholipid syndrome (APS) is, usually, both easily confirmed with readily available blood tests (antiphospholipid antibodies/"aPL") and successfully treated – sometimes with as basic a medicine as "baby" aspirin.

Although our repertoire of useful drugs is limited (aspirin, heparin, warfarin), one important lesson has been that with very careful management, such as ensuring that the warfarin dose is adequate, spectacular results can be obtained.

In this short work, I hope to present, with the help of 50 illustrative case reports, a patients' perspective.

An extract from the original description appears as an appendix at the end of this volume.

Section I
The Brain

Though the dull brain perplexes and retards.

(Keats. Ode to a Nightingale. 1820)

… If the brain does not get its normal supply of circulation, and of oxygen, its protests, as you will read, can take many forms…

CASE I
Late for the Wedding......

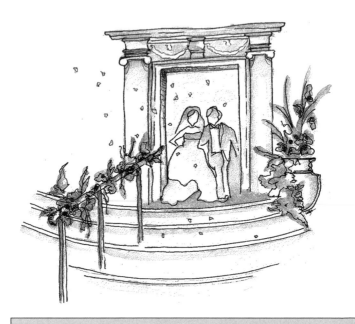

- Loss of speech
- Headaches
- Encephalitis look-alike

H.C., a 21-year-old, was due to marry on Saturday. For 2 weeks before the wedding, she complained of fatigue, headaches and poor concentration. The symptoms were attributed to stress and she battled on.

On the morning of the wedding, she became more unwell – at first vague and withdrawn, but soon, clearly not right. Dramatically, she became mute – could not speak.

An ambulance was called and she was seen in hospital emergency, where an initial diagnosis of hysteria was seriously considered. However, the neurologist who was called in found a number of surprisingly abnormal neurological signs – indeed; he concluded that here was a girl with widespread severe neurological disease – possibly encephalitis.

Here, the story took an important twist. One of the junior doctors wondered if she had a face rash suggestive of lupus (the "butterfly" rash). And so it turned out. She was treated with steroids and other drugs and slowly, over a period of months, she improved.

Comment

Twenty-five years on, H.C. still attends the lupus clinic. Her antiphospholipid (aPL) antibodies, first measured 4 years after the initial dramatic illness, remain strongly positive. The patient herself is well, with slightly raised blood pressure, and prominent skin blotchiness (livedo reticularis). She takes aspirin daily together with her various alternative medicines but resolutely declines any thought of warfarin or other "poisonous" drugs. So far, she is proving to be correct.

In retrospect, her dramatic presentation was much more likely to have been due to antiphospholipid syndrome (APS) than to the lupus. Her improvement, had the condition been known, might have been far more speedy with anticoagulants.

Up to two in five patients with lupus carry aPL antibodies. As in this case, the underlying lupus may be mild, but the clotting tendency associated with aPL can be devastating.

Take Home Message

The brain can be profoundly affected if its blood supply is compromised…

Hughes syndrome is one such compromise.

CASE 2
Falling Over ......

- Drop attacks
- A form of epilepsy?
- Response to warfarin

There are some medical cases that seem to defy explanation. Yet they are very real.

Mrs. L.J., aged 47, had suffered from mild lupus – diagnosed in her 30s, and well controlled on simple antimalarials (hydroxychloroquine). Her previous symptoms had included sun-sensitive rashes and aches and pains.

For the past 2 years, she had suffered from what she quite simply described as "falling over". One moment she would be walking – in a shop, down the road, in her garden – and the next she would have "fallen over" – witnessed as a sudden "drop attack" – seconds only, and with no seizures or other epileptic features. There were no headaches or warnings. She would simply shake herself and get up again.

Otherwise, she was well. Perhaps, during the past 2 years there had been some memory loss – well, possibly more than she wanted to admit.

Attending the lupus clinic, Mrs. L.J. was found to have positive aPL tests but had no previous history of thrombosis or miscarriage. However, in view of this, the memory loss and the odd "falling over" history an electro-encephalogram (EEG) and an magnetic resonance imaging (MRI) were carried out. These showed abnormal electrical waves and numerous unidentified bright objects (UBOs) – small white dots – almost certainly due to poor circulation and small clots. It was decided to go for a trial of warfarin anticoagulation. There was a complete and sustained end to the "falling over" episodes. At the same time, the patient was delighted in the improvement of her memory and in her general "sharpness".

Comment

In retrospect, this patient was suffering from significant brain clotting, as evidenced by the abnormal MRI and the improvement on warfarin.

In this patient, the attacks were almost certainly a form of epilepsy – now recognized as an important feature in some patients with Hughes syndrome.

Such has been the importance of this discovery that neurologists are beginning to re-study some of their patients with epilepsy for evidence of "sticky blood." And the results are interesting: a recent study from Milan found that one in five of "idiopathic" (i.e. without an obvious cause such as head injury), teenage epileptics had positive aPL tests.

Take Home Message
Hughes syndrome can cause seizures.

CASE 3
Diplomatic Epilepsy......

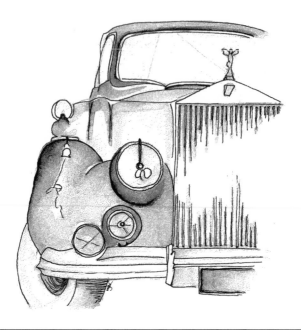

- Mild lupus...but...
- ...very severe epilepsy
- "Sticky blood"
- Warfarin: epilepsy better

The following case represents the more severe end of the "epilepsy spectrum."

A 42-year-old wife of an American diplomat had a past history of lupus, now well controlled on a small dose of steroids (5 mg prednisolone daily). Her major problem, and one with a major impact on her busy life, was recurrent seizures – both petit mal and grand mal, for which she had received a variety of combinations of anti-epileptic treatment. On examination, the only abnormality was a blotchy skin appearance known as livedo reticularis. Blood tests showed the lupus to be inactive, but she had extremely high levels of aPL antibodies. During her stay in London, she developed a deep vein thrombosis (DVT) of the leg and routine anticoagulation with *warfarin (Coumadin) was started. An immediate and unexpected bonus was a marked reduction in frequency and severity of the seizures – requiring far less aggressive anti-epileptic treatment.*

Comment

The brain's list of responses to insult is limited. One of the most dramatic is with fits or seizures. All types of fits have been described, including petit mal ("absences"), temporal lobe epilepsy (with its unusual characteristics such as "déjà vu") and grand mal (seizures).

In most cases, the fits are limited to a first or major event, and recurrent fits are thought to be uncommon, though, as in the previous case, it is possible that the full association is under-recognized.

It is difficult to explain the improvement following anticoagulation in a problem which has been long-standing. Nevertheless, that is what happened. In this, as in other cases with clear improvement with blood–thinning medicines, it may be that "sludging" of the blood rather than irreversible clotting, is the predominant mechanism.

Take Home Message

A new and potentially treatable cause of epilepsy has been described in this patient's case.

This patient had epilepsy with recurrent seizures (both petit mal and grand mal), livedo reticularis and finally DVT which when treated with anticoagulants, helped improve her long time endured epilepsy.

CASE 4
Weak Legs ......

- Spinal cord...
- Walking affected...
- Bladder control poor
- Improvement with treatment

(The following two cases were dramatic, with involvement of the spinal cord).

James, a 30-year-old marketing businessman, started to complain of leg weakness. At first, he put it down to "ageing" but, over the course of a few months, found that on certain days, he had real difficulty in walking. His general practitioner (GP) referred him to a neurologist who suspected a problem in the spinal cord – possibly "myelopathy" or perhaps a form of multiple sclerosis (MS).

An MRI scan showed no abnormality, but with increasing weakness, and the first suggestions of a problem with bladder control, repeat MRI showed abnormalities in the spinal cord.

Although a working diagnosis of "MS" was made, James turned out to be one of the "fortunate" early cases to be diagnosed as APS with marked improvement in warfarin treatment. He is now stable with no progression of the disease over an 8-year period.

Comment
Mention the spinal cord, the brain, balance and vision problems and the possible diagnosis of MS is raised. MS is common, and takes many clinical forms. The similarities between Hughes syndrome and MS can be striking.

Some years ago, we published a detailed study of a group of patients with Hughes syndrome who had originally been considered to have "MS."

There were a number of conclusions – some sobering:

The two conditions could be clinically indistinguishable. The MRIs were often indistinguishable. Notably, however, in those patients ultimately diagnosed as Hughes syndrome and treated with warfarin, there was no further deterioration.

Take Home Message
Some cases of "MS" may in fact have Hughes syndrome.

The similarities between MS and Hughes syndrome are striking. Research is currently underway to examine the possibility of misdiagnosis in some patients with MS .

This patient showed progressive weakness, abnormalities to the spinal cord shown on MRI, difficulty walking and bladder control all pointing to MS but for one fortunate difference, that his blood test indicated Hughes syndrome. Not only did he get better with warfarin – 8 years later he has not had any further deterioration.

CASE 5
"Multiple Sclerosis" ......

- ...can mimic MS
- Diagnosis after DVT
- Simple blood test for Hughes syndrome

A 23-year-old neurophysiology student developed headaches, occasional movement disorders, slight difficulty with gait and visual disturbance. Brain scanning (MRI) showed two small lesions, and a diagnosis of "possible MS" was made. The student's future was uncertain. She also went on to develop a low platelet count in the blood, a possible thrombosis in the leg and increasing migraines. She was found to be aPL positive, and the diagnosis was changed to Hughes syndrome. Following the leg DVT, she was anticoagulated and has remained well since. There have been no new neurological features in 5 years' follow-up.

Comment
What is the extent of the "overlap" between Hughes syndrome and MS? Are there any clinical clues which might help distinguish? In a recent patient audit in our clinic, we asked all our patients the same question... "Did your doctor(s) at any stage mention the possible diagnosis of MS?" Nearly one-third (32%) of aPL – positive patients answered "yes" compared with 8% of controls.

Clearly, there are patients attending MS clinics who may well have a different condition – Hughes syndrome. Whether the figure is 1%, 5% or more, or less, is not known and it will take very careful studies in large neurology clinics before we know.

As to the second question, there are some clinical clues. For example, I have suggested a 4-point questionnaire which might point more towards Hughes syndrome.

1. Have you ever had a thrombosis (e.g., a DVT)?
2. If ever pregnant, have you had a miscarriage?
3. Have you suffered migraine or severe headaches? (more a feature of Hughes syndrome than MS)
4. Do you have a family history of autoimmune disease such as lupus, thyroid disease or rheumatoid arthritis (commoner in Hughes syndrome)

Although these questions might provide "soft" data, I am optimistic that with greater recognition of APS, and with better brain scanning techniques and more sensitive blood tests, this important clinical question will be resolved.

Take Home Message
Hughes syndrome – potentially treatable – can mimic MS. Therefore, it is always worth blood testing!

We are still some way from knowing how many patients attending MS clinics around the world have Hughes syndrome.

CASE 6

Teenage Migraine.......

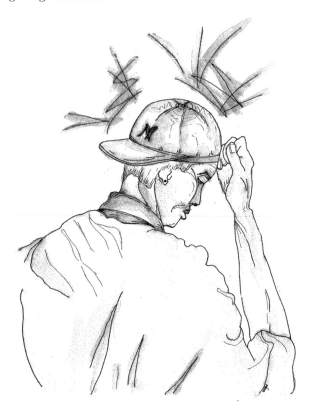

- Migraine and miscarriages...
- ...think Hughes syndrome
- Successful pregnancy with aspirin

*A 14-year-old girl complained of frequent headaches – often pre-
cipitated by stress and school examinations. These headaches were
frequently migrainous, with "flashing lights" and nausea, and for
a period of about 3 years, she would miss 3–4 days of school each
month. At times, the migraines were severe enough to affect speech
and to cause weakness in the arms and legs. A medical label of
"hemiplegic migraine" was put forward and a variety of migraine
pills prescribed.*

In her 20s, the problem settled. Between the ages of 25 and 30, she suffered several miscarriages. A blood test showed positive for aPL antibodies . She was treated with daily aspirin and subsequently had two successful pregnancies.

Comment

Headache is one of the cardinal features of Hughes syndrome. Many, many patients complain of headache – often migrainous, and often in childhood and the teens.

In many cases, the migraine seems to run in the family. Sometimes the headaches disappear in the 20s, only to return later.

Testing for aPL in the blood is simple and cheap. As so many Hughes syndrome patients with headaches improve with blood-thinning agents (aspirin, clopidogrel, heparin or warfarin) screening for Hughes syndrome seems a worthwhile exercise (Fig. 6.1).

Hughes Syndrome Patients' Questionnaire Fig. 6.1

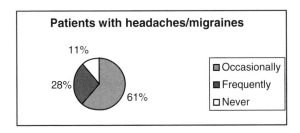

Take Home Message

Migraine is common in Hughes syndrome. A simple, inexpensive blood test could be critical.

As seen in this patient's story, migraines can be so severe that they can affect speech, vision and weakness in the arms and legs. After several miscarriages, a blood test was performed and was positive for Hughes syndrome. Then given proper medication, she went on to have two healthy babies.

CASE 7
Getting Only Half the Picture

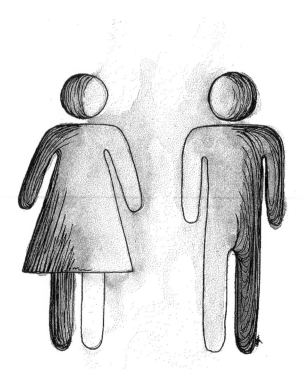

- Eye symptoms common
- Visual field loss

Mrs. A.D., a busy shop owner, had been previously well, when at the age of 34, she started complaining of headaches – at first weekly (and worse before her periods) but later, daily. During one exceptionally severe headache, she found that her vision had been affected. In fact, she was unable to see the right side of her field of vision (she was later able to joke that she would often walk into the lad's instead of the ladies). She was referred to a neurologist who diagnosed a slight stroke. However, the brain scan (MRI) was normal. No obvious precipitating factors were found, but she was started on daily low-dose aspirin. Some years later, she was found to have positive aPL tests.

Comment

The visual fields are mapped out in the brain. Blood clots or other lesions affecting either this part of the brain or the nervous system circuits from the retina of the eye to the brain can result in a cut-off of the field of vision, sometimes a loss of one quarter, or even one-half of the field of vision

This symptom, often known as "hemianopia" has been a clinical feature in a number of patients with "sticky blood."

It could be argued that in this patient's case, despite the negative brain scan, this was almost certainly a result of a brain clot, and that warfarin would be a better option – more likely to prevent future stroke (Fig. 7.1).

Hughes Syndrome Patients' Questionnaire Fig. 7.1

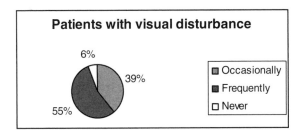

Patients with visual disturbance

6%
39%
55%

- ▨ Occasionally
- ▧ Frequently
- ☐ Never

Take Home Message

Loss of a part of the field of vision could be due to blood clotting in the brain.

CASE 8
Difficult Crossword Puzzles......

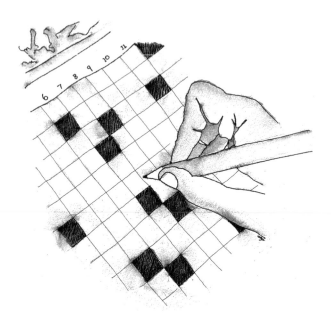

- Memory loss important
- NOT Alzheimer's
- Can improve with treatment

Mrs. T.J., aged 51, had suffered for 1–2 years from increasingly severe headaches. She had visited her doctor but no obvious cause had been found. To rule out a brain tumour, she underwent an MRI which was normal. Her past history was significant in that she had suffered severely from teenage headaches and had had 2 (or possibly 3) miscarriages.

Further investigation demonstrated high levels of aPL. She was started on aspirin with some (incomplete) improvement in headaches.

Over the next year, it became clear that her memory loss was giving cause for concern. At first, this was a private "joke" within the family. However, serious worries about the possibility of Alzheimer's disease were raised.

Mrs. J., who normally completed the newspaper crossword every day of her life in 15 minutes, now, for example, would take up to 1 hour agonizing over the clues.

A brain scan on this occasion showed one or two small "dots." In view of the known diagnosis of Hughes syndrome, she was referred to our clinic, where it was decided to start warfarin.

Like so many patients before her, Mrs. J. described her improvement as a "mist lifting". She felt mentally "sharp" and, at last the headaches finally cleared.

Formal memory testing in our unit (part of our clinical evaluation) showed striking improvement in all memory and "cognitive" tests.

Perhaps the most tellingly, she was now back to the standard 15 minutes for the crossword.

Comment

This patient provides an interesting anecdote. Like so many others, she "knew" when the warfarin control was correct. If the INR (international normalized ratio) (see later) fell below 3 and the blood became "sticky" again, she took longer over the crossword.

The patient has provided me, at my request, with a wonderful graph showing the absolute correlation between the INR (which she self-tests) and "crossword puzzle time" – as sophisticated an observation as any complicated "psychometric" test.[1]

Take Home Message

Many patients with Hughes syndrome suffer memory problems. With treatment, improvement can be striking.

---

[1] Here, again is an example of a 50-something year old with one or two small 'lesions' on MRI. Conventional teaching might have accepted these as part of the 'normal' ageing process. Not so.

CASE 9
Playing the Wrong Notes ......

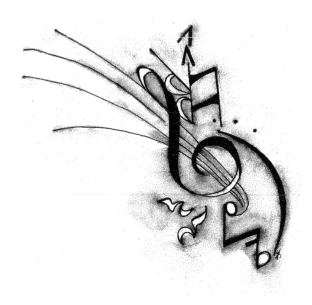

> • Skin mottling – "livedo reticularis" ("corned beef skin")
> • Very important clue

I suppose that in choosing case reports, there is a natural tendency to report successes rather than failures. The next case definitely qualifies as a failure!

The 52-year-old pianist in a traveling South African "3-man" band had started to make mistakes at the piano. At first these were ignored and finally, sadly, she had to give up her place in the band. Over the next year, she became clearly more disabled, with slurring of words, giddiness, severe memory problems and difficulty in walking.

Neurological examination showed multiple abnormalities including loss of part of the field of vision. There was severe cognitive impairment. The skin showed florid, blotchy "livedo reticularis." A brain scan showed widespread, severe brain lesions.

Investigations were negative for the known causes of widespread brain disease, but she was positive for aPL, both by the anticardiolipin and by the lupus anticoagulant tests.

She was diagnosed with Hughes syndrome and started on warfarin, maintaining a high INR. Although she felt some improvement, her neurological problems and memory defect remained severe.

Comment

Here is the extreme end of the "neurological" spectrum of Hughes syndrome, ranking with the worst cases of AIDS, of Mad Cow Disease, or of any other cause of severe brain pathology.

Our papers on Hughes syndrome in the early 1980s included cases of "dementia." In the patient described here, it is sadly unlikely whether warfarin will result in much improvement.

Think of what an earlier diagnosis might have achieved.

Picking up the earliest clinical clues such as memory impairment and having the confidence to treat firmly – with warfarin anticoagulation if need be – could prove to be the single most positive aspect of the whole "antiphospholipid" story.

Take Home Message

The danger in Hughes syndrome is clotting (NOT bleeding). This case puts the strongest argument for early treatment.

This is one of the most severe patients in these case studies presenting with symptoms including slurring of words, giddiness, severe memory problems, difficulty in walking and loss of part of the field of vision.

CASE 10
Speaking Gibberish ......

- Speech disturbance
- "TIA's" and strokes
- Treatment urgent

A 26-year old previously fit building laborer became unwell at a railway station whilst going to a sports fixture with friends. He suffered a headache and, according to his friends, started "speaking gibberish." The speech disturbance lasted 15 minutes. On admission to hospital, he had slight weakness on one side of the face. His brain scan was normal and he made a full recovery. He remembered suffering a similar but less severe episode 3 months previously. He was found to be aPL positive and was subsequently treated with warfarin (Coumadin).

Comment
Scanning techniques have helped in diagnosis. The MRI scan is the most widely used. Areas of brain damage due to a lack of oxygen show up as white areas ("dots"), varying in size from the pinprick to larger prominent areas (Fig. 10.1). In some patients, the MRI resembles the sky at night.

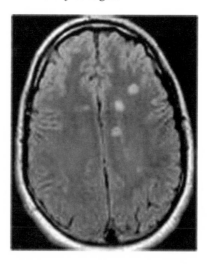

FIG. 10.1. Brain MRI scan showing lesions (white dots)

For doctors and patients dealing with Hughes syndrome, while the MRI scan of the brain (and spinal cord) is the best available test of brain injury, it is not "perfect," and, as in the case of this patient, who clearly suffered a "TIA" (transient ischemic attack), the results are often negative. Newer techniques such as the "PET" (positron emission tomography) scan are being developed but are not yet available for widespread clinical use.

Take Home Message
A young person with stroke-like symptoms of speaking gibberish and partial facial paralysis: think Hughes syndrome. Potentially treatable.

CASE 11
I Lost My Sense of Smell ......

- Loss of smell
- ...is seen in some brain conditions
- Possibly uncommon

A 60-year-old lady developed acute stiffness of the shoulder girdles, low back and hips. She was diagnosed as having the acute (and treatable) rheumatic condition called "polymyalgia" and responded well to treatment.

At the same time as the rheumatic illness, she developed memory problems and the sudden loss of the sense of smell. Blood tests showed medium high levels of aPL.

Five years later, she remains perfectly well (on aspirin) but with no return of the sense of smell. The aPL antibodies have disappeared.

Comment
Polymyalgia rheumatica, an acute musculo-rheumatic condition, usually responds to a course of steroids. However, it can cause neurological features and is one of the few medical conditions which have been occasionally seen to produce aPL – the antibodies disappearing with time.

This patient is one of a small number attending my clinic, who have developed the sudden loss of the sense of smell (anosmia) – a condition well recognized by neurologists (Fig. 11.1).

Hughes Syndrome Patients' Questionnaire Fig. 11.1

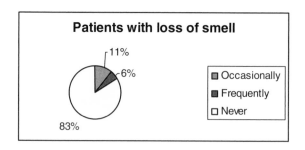

Take Home Message
Loss of sense of smell can be a lesser-known result of a brain insult – possibly, in this case, due to "sticky blood."

CASE 12
Movement, Jerks and Twitches ......

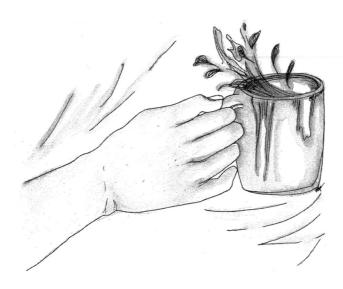

- Jerks, tics, twitches...
- ...all types of movement disorder

A 53-year-old secretary developed a marked sudden twitching movement in her right arm. Some months later, there was a similar, poorly controlled twitching in the face muscles.

The arm jerks – sometimes severe enough to throw water out of a glass – became sufficiently severe for her to have to leave her job. She was investigated by my neurology colleagues, whose findings included a strongly positive anticardiolipin test. Treatment with anticoagulants produced a marked improvement – though not a complete disappearance of the jerking movements.

Comment
Another way in which the brain expresses its dislike of poor circulation is with movement disorders. These can vary from mild occasional twitches through to writhing movements (St. Vitus Dance) – and even more.

Take Home Message

Jerks and movement disorders are some of the ways in which the brain "protests."

(Neurologists now recognize a wide variety of "movement disorders" in Hughes syndrome – though none as dramatic as our next case.)

CASE 13
Mad Cow Disease ......

- Extreme brain involvement...
- ...can also respond to treatment

A 53-year-old farmer's wife developed twitching movements, gradually worsening over a 9-month period. At first, individual muscle groups were affected, but gradually the limbs, the trunk and the head were affected.

Extensive neurological investigation did not come to a firm conclusion, but the weight of opinion was that this was most probably a case of "variant C.J.D" (Creutzfeld-Jacob disease) – more colloquially known as "mad cow disease." The prognosis was poor.

The investigations turned up one surprise – an astronomically high level of anticardiolipin antibody – perhaps not such a surprise as the patient's past history included two previous miscarriages and a possible DVT.

It seemed a long shot, but the neurologists decided that there might be a link. Warfarin was worth a try. Nothing to lose.

The result is history. The movements lessened, the patient improved and, at the time of writing, 8 years after the start of treatment, remains well. Interestingly, her condition requires strong anticoagulation – when the INR falls below 3.4 the twitching returns.

Comment
An extreme example of the potential impact of Hughes syndrome on the central nervous system – and a perfect example of the need for very precise control of warfarin dosage. Little use this patient following the average anticoagulation control of INR 1.5–2!

Blood thinning needs to be precise: think of the analogy of supermarket milk – An INR of 1.5 = slightly less-cream milk. An INR of 2–2.5 = semi-skimmed milk. An INR of 3 or over = skimmed milk.

Take Home Message
Another extreme example of "sticky blood." Like the car engine which stutters when the mixture of petrol/gas is wrong, the brain is exquisitely sensitive to a sludging of the blood supply.

CASE 14
St. Vitus Dance ......

> • Once common in rheumatic fever
> • Now seen in Hughes syndrome
> • Improves with blood thinning

A peculiar movement disorder, known as chorea or St. Vitus Dance, was found during the last century to be an unusual feature of rheumatic fever. Patients would develop writhing arm movements, reminiscent of the arm and finger movements of Balinese or Thai dancers.

Although the most well-known cause of chorea is rheumatic fever (due to a streptococcal infection), other causes, notably lupus, have been associated, especially when the oral contraceptive pill is started.

In 1983, we reported that aPL antibodies were associated with St. Vitus Dance. Since then, so many cases have been reported that it is possible that Hughes syndrome is now a commoner cause of chorea than rheumatic fever.

A 26-year-old woman with a known history of lupus developed repetitive movements, especially of the arms. The movements, diagnosed as chorea, persisted for many months. There was no improvement with a short course of steroids.

As so often seems to be the case in this series of case reports, fate took a hand. The patient developed an acute vein thrombosis in the leg and was commenced on warfarin. There was a rapid and clear cut improvement in the chorea. Her aPL tests were strongly positive.

Comment
It is difficult to explain the improvement in chorea associated with warfarin treatment. A perhaps simplistic explanation might be the improvement in "sludging" of the brain circulation with thinning of the blood.

It may also be coincidence. However, chorea is a fairly rare medical condition and it did not take long for numerous similar reports associating Hughes syndrome with chorea to appear.

It is also interesting that chorea has been described in association with the oral contraceptive pill – something in common with a number of Hughes syndrome features such as headache and thrombosis.

Take Home Message
Some cases of St. Vitus' Dance – and other movement disorders – may be attributable to Hughes syndrome. And treatable.

CASE 15
Parkinson's Disease ......

- Parkinson tremor sometimes seen
- Low platelet counts a clue

This – one of the commoner forms of neurological tremor, has also, intriguingly, been linked in some cases of Hughes syndrome.

While this series of cases perhaps understandably focuses on success, the following case, at the time of writing, has not had such an outcome.

Mrs. A.Y., aged 59, had been known to suffer from Hughes syndrome (with positive aPL) for 18 years. Her history included headaches, and difficulties in word finding, but most chronically, of low platelets with counts usually between 50,000 and 70,000 (the normal platelet count is over 150,000). Occasionally, the platelet count would fall precipitously and require a short course of steroids. Despite these problems, she lived a full and active life.

For the past 2 years, she has developed a rapidly progressive "ball rolling" tremor of the hands as well as other clinical features of Parkinsonism, not at present well controlled on anti-Parkinson medication.

She is on aspirin, has a normal brain scan, and has never had a thrombosis.

Comment
Would you consider other drugs? Although she has never had clinical thrombosis, the lessons from other neurological diseases associated with aPL would suggest a trial of either heparin or warfarin. The patient is, at present, against these medicines. But, watch this space!

Take Home Message
As with MS, stroke, memory loss, migraine – all common conditions – a small percentage of cases of Parkinson's disease might be due to (reversible) "sticky blood."

CASE 16
Missing the Target ......

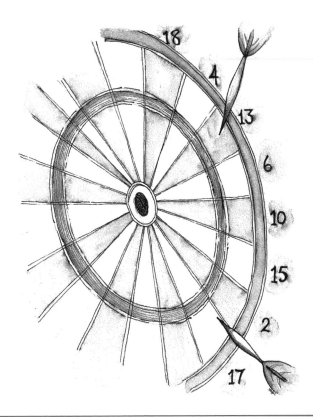

- "Mini-clots" in brain
- Effects can be very localized

A 40-year-old woman, the champion of her country village darts team, suddenly became unable to "hit the 20" – she could not recognize its number or position. She was found to have APS and, on brain scan, had one small area of clot.

Comment
Darts, a game of skill played around the world, but especially traditional in the English country pub, is a game of skill, requiring hand–eye coordination – and an intact wiring circuit through the

brain. This case is an example of the occasionally very specific defect caused by a small brain lesion – presumably a small clot.

Take Home Message
An example of a "wiring problem" (loss of hand and eye coordination) in the brain resulting from a mini-stroke in untreated Hughes syndrome (Fig. 16.1).

From "focal" lesion to more "generalized" brain lesion – the following important case illustrates the need for correct diagnosis.

Hughes Syndrome Patients' Questionnaire Fig. 16.1

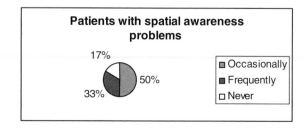

CASE 17
The Headmistress Who Forgot ......

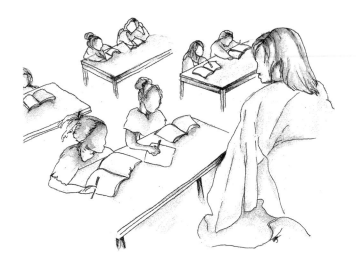

- Memory loss changes lives
- Potentially reversible in Hughes syndrome

A highly successful 52-year-old school head-teacher at one of London's leading schools, started to complain of memory loss, fatigue and a lack of drive and energy. There were occasional headaches. She was investigated but no diagnosis was made. A course of antidepressants was unhelpful. She was unable to continue in her job. Three years later, she developed a stroke, thought initially to be due to a brain hemorrhage, but subsequently thought to be due to a blood clot. It was soon after this that she was found to have positive aPL. After discussion, it was decided to start warfarin. The result was dramatic. There was a disappearance of the mental sluggishness and fatigue, and a return to a reasonably normal life. Like many other patients, she "knows" precisely when the anticoagulant control ("INR") has slipped – the headaches and "foggy–brain" return.

Comment
This case report underlines I believe, the importance of diagnosis and correct management of the syndrome. The brain features, whilst often subtle enough to go undiagnosed, are devastating for the patient who suffers them. All too often it is possible to

attribute treatable organic disease such as this to "depression," or the "menopause" or "stress".

Take Home Message
Listen to the patient.

CASE 18
"Personality Disorder" in a 4-Year-Old ......

- Children too!
- ... "personality disorder"

A 4-year-old boy was referred from Italy for advice regarding management. He had developed a marked personality disorder, with aggressive behavior, poor memory and with one seizure. Investigations revealed multiple lesions, especially in the frontal (front) cortex area of the brain. He was aPL positive. He has been started on warfarin – probably for life.

Comment
Hughes syndrome is most commonly diagnosed after the age of 20 (possibly with a bias brought about by the more widespread testing in pregnancy). However, the disease *is* recognized in children and even in infants.

In addition to the well-recognized association with epilepsy and seizure, this case suggests that brain involvement in children with Hughes syndrome can present with "neuro-psychiatric" manifestations. My own practice includes two patients with Hughes syndrome patients with obsessive–compulsive disorder (OCD) who improved with anticoagulation treatment.

Take Home Message
Although Hughes syndrome is rarely found in children, brain discomfort can take the form of psychiatric problems (personality disorder, aggressive behavior and poor memory) as well as neurologic features such as seizures.

CASE 19
To Sleep ... Perchance to Dream

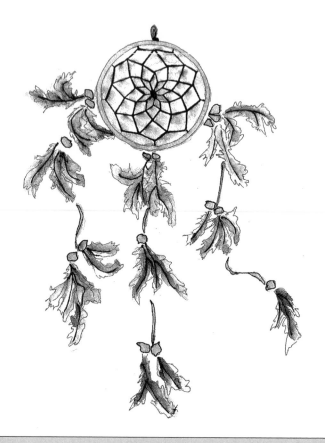

- Frequency of sleep disturbance unknown
- Some cases of narcolepsy seen

A number of patients with Hughes syndrome complain bitterly of sleep disturbance.

A 38-year-old patient with a diagnosis of Hughes syndrome (previous DVT, miscarriage, headaches) was doing reasonably well on aspirin alone. However, her sleep pattern was seriously disturbed. As well as finding sleep a problem at night, she began to suffer bizarre sleep problems during the day, sometimes falling asleep at odd times of the day, often totally unexpectedly. She was investigated by a specialist sleep centre and found to have severely abnormal sleep patterns. Treatment by various medications has helped, but sleep disturbance has been a problem. She has been treated with aspirin, but, as distinct from some of our other patients with Hughes syndrome and sleep disorder, improvement has been disappointing.

Comment

A number of patients have had sleep disturbance, some with full-blown narcolepsy. Our team is currently undertaking a combined study of these patients with our sleep research centre. Presumably, like so many of the other features seen in the cases reported here, it is yet another manifestation of the brain protesting against an impaired blood and oxygen supply.

Take Home Message

Narcolepsy and sleep disturbance. APS may represent a newly recognized cause. The ripples of the syndrome spread wider (Fig. 19.1).

Hughes Syndrome Patients' Questionnaire Fig. 19.1

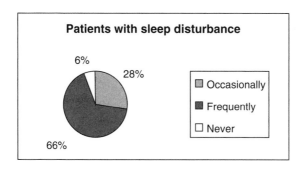

Patients with sleep disturbance

6%
28%
66%

☐ Occasionally
■ Frequently
☐ Never

Section 2
........and Other Organs

Like the brain, all other organs of the body are critically dependent on a good oxygen supply. Even a minimal reduction, such as that caused by "sticky blood," can have potentially devastating effects ... effects which could be totally prevented by correct diagnosis and treatment.

CASE 20
The Lung

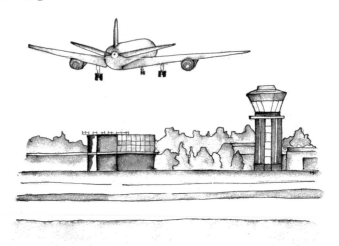

Collapse at the Airport ......

- Lung clots ("pulmonary embolism")
- Often follow leg or pelvic clots
- Increased risk in Hughes syndrome

A 42-year-old business woman returned to London on an overnight flight from Los Angeles. She had been previously well and had had an uneventful flight. She had drunk one glass of wine on the plane, and had "topped up" with water.

On arrival at Heathrow airport, she made her way off the plane at the usual snail's pace with the rest of the passengers. As she walked up the connecting gangway into the airport, she felt giddy, suddenly unwell and short of breath. She managed to hold on to a pillar, but then collapsed. She was taken to the medical centre at the airport and transferred to hospital as an emergency.

The diagnosis was, in fact, a "pulmonary embolism" – a lung blood clot. Although there was no clear proof, it was suspected that the clot had arisen in one of the leg or pelvic veins and traveled onto the lung.

She was treated in intensive care, and ultimately made a full recovery. Subsequent tests revealed high levels of aCL and long-term anticoagulants were advised.

Comment

A survey at a hospital close to Charles de Gaulle airport in Paris showed that a peak danger time for "PE" (lung blood clot) was the period between leaving the aeroplane and reaching the arrivals lounge. One theory suggests that the leg or pelvic clot forms during the immobility of the long flight, and that the unstable clot breaks loose when the person gets up and starts moving.

Whatever the theory, the risk of blood clots during or after long air (and other) journeys has become widely trumpeted, the term "economy class syndrome" being something of a cause celebre in the media and amongst the more litigiously minded.

The thrombosis risks are well known – stress, immobility, alcohol, dehydration and the airlines are cooperating in publicizing these risks.

However, there are undoubtedly some individuals, such as the patient described here, in whom other, "hidden" risk factors are present. One such risk factor could well be antiphospholipid antibodies (aPL) – certainly at least worth taking a precautionary aspirin before a long flight. A number of my patients with antiphospholipid syndrome (APS) on long-term aspirin take a single injection of heparin for flights of 8 hours or more. While there are no definitive studies of this aspect of treatment, there is certainly some logic in it.

Take Home Message

Pulmonary embolism (a "clot on the lung") is one of medicine's great emergencies, and a major cause of sudden death in both old and young.

This case illustrates the importance of screening for "at risk" individuals such as those with Hughes syndrome.

CASE 21
The Skin

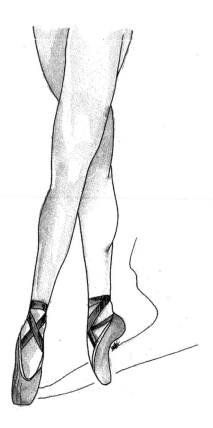

Ballerina's Leg Ulcers ......

- Leg ulcers can follow leg clots
- Can improve with blood-thinning

A 34-year-old Latvian ballerina's career was cut short by a sudden leg thrombosis (deep vein thrombosis, DVT), followed by a second in the other leg soon after her 6 months' course of warfarin was stopped.

Following a second course of warfarin, she remained well apart from the development of discolored skin on both shins – attributed to the old DVTs. Unfortunately, over a period of 1–2 years, areas of the skin broke down, and the patient developed a number of chronic, very painful, ulcers on the lower part of the legs. Her ballet career came to a sudden stop.

She was admitted to hospital where investigations showed positive aPL tests. The patient was started on long-term warfarin. With time the ulcers slowly healed.

Over the next 2 years, an interesting observation was made: on the two occasions when the warfarin was stopped, the ulcers quickly returned, improving only when the warfarin was restarted.

Comment

Chronic leg ulcers are a feared complication of leg vein thrombosis. They are common and often slow to heal. Hospital beds throughout the world have long-stay patients with leg ulcer in them.

The observation that post-thrombotic leg ulcers in patients with Hughes syndrome might respond more quickly with anti-coagulation could have important consequences in this difficult condition.

To date, no major study of the prevalence of Hughes syndrome in a large leg ulcer clinic population has been attempted.

Take Home Message
There are a number of causes of chronic leg ulcers. Hughes syndrome – "sticky blood" – a potentially treatable condition – is one of them.

CASE 22
The Liver

Twenty Years On ......

• Liver clots can occur
• Always check liver tests in Hughes syndrome

Miss M.R., a 16-year-old law student from Lisbon, developed leg thrombosis on starting the oral contraceptive pill. Her condition worsened and she developed shortness of breath (thought to be due to a lung clot or "pulmonary embolism") and jaundice. Investigations showed that she had developed widespread clotting in the veins of the liver. The circulation of the skin of the legs became poor and she developed a number of leg ulcers.

She was sent to London for a second opinion. Her anticardiolipin levels were extremely high (this was at the time in the early 1980s when we were publishing our methods for measuring aPL).

She was started on warfarin, maintaining an international normalized ratio (INR) of 3 or more, and gradually over a year or so, the ulcers healed. The liver tests returned to normal and the patient returned to her normal life.

Over the next 20 years, the patient has maintained a precise and careful watch on her INR. She found, early on, that a prolonged fall in the INR brought back the leg ulcers.

Twenty years on, aged 36, the patient is a busy and successful lawyer and housewife. Her anticardiolipin levels remain high. Her liver function tests are normal.

Comment
This patient teaches us a number of lessons. The liver, like every other organ, can be affected by blood clotting – indeed one study in America suggests that APS is now one of the leading causes of the liver clotting disease known as Budd-Chiari syndrome.

Secondly, despite the severe degree of liver thrombosis, anticoagulant treatment, as well as time, has shown liver healing.

Thirdly, the post-thrombosis leg ulcers appear to be sensitive to the correct level of anticoagulation (INR).

Take Home Message
This young lady is one of my early 1980s patients. Twenty years on, she leads a busy life – but in her particular case, the antibody is still there, and to stop the treatment now would be wrong. It could cause recurrence of liver disease, leg ulcers, DVTs, or pulmonary embolism.

CASE 23
The Heart

"Heart Attack"

- Arteries can clot
- …e.g. coronary arteries
- An important cause of heart attack?

A 46-year-old housewife developed chest pains, later diagnosed as angina. Her previous history included teenage migraine, and previous investigation for "multiple sclerosis," with features including severe visual disturbance, giddiness, numbness and memory loss.

One morning, she developed severe chest pains and was admitted to the intensive care ward with a heart attack. Emergency treatment included heparin. An interesting observation was made by the patient: within 2 days of heparin injections … "to my amazement I could read, my eyes were totally clear."

A year later she had a severe angina attack. Hospital tests confirmed the unstable angina, but surprisingly showed wide open, clear coronary arteries (sometimes known in cardiology circles as "Syndrome X"). At this time she was found to have anticardiolipin antibodies.

She was finally treated on long term warfarin, with disappearance not only of her chest pains but also of her distressing visual and neurological symptoms.

Comment
The brief summary is taken from the history of one of my patients Mrs. Kay Thackray whose biographical book "Sticky Blood Explained"[1] is the best description I have read of the trials, tribulations and courage needed, in a patient with a complicated, and "new" disease. I think it should be essential reading for all patients and doctors involved with this disease.

Take Home Message
The heart, like the brain, can be susceptible to "sticky blood."

---

[1] Sticky Blood Explained. Kay Thackray – 2002 J R Digital Print services Ltd. ISBN 1898030774

CASE 24

Backpacking in Australia

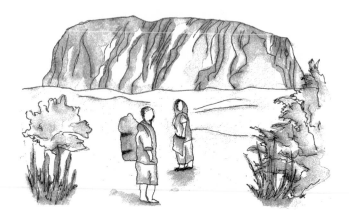

- How common is Hughes syndrome in "young" heart attacks
- A major need for more research

A 23-year-old college student had previously been diagnosed as having mild lupus. She had also been found to have strongly positive aPL and was taking baby aspirin daily. The lupus was asymptomatic, the tests were good and she was on no other therapy.

Half way through a backpacking holiday in Australia, she developed severe chest pain and collapsed. She was taken to hospital but attempts to resuscitate her failed. She was pronounced dead some 3 hours after the onset of chest pain.

At post-mortem, she was found to have a major coronary artery thrombosis – a heart attack. There were no other significant findings.

Comment

This tragic case highlights the extreme, life-threatening end of Hughes syndrome: the fact that arteries can clot as well as veins. It also highlights a number of questions.

- Is aspirin sufficient protection? Certainly not in this case.
- What other risk factors are present? No obvious ones in this case. Neither the weather nor the exercise was extreme.
- Could Hughes syndrome be a factor in other cases of "unexplained" heart attacks? The answer is almost certainly *yes*.

At long last, a number of studies are being reported looking at aPL in cardiology clinics. A recent study, for example, found that over 20% of young women (under 31) with heart attack were aPL positive – an observation of huge importance.

Take Home Message
Maybe aPL testing will one day assume the importance in preventative medicine that cholesterol now enjoys in the fight against heart disease.

CASE 25

Short of Breath in Scandinavia ......

- Heart valves can be affected
- Heart murmurs
- Valve failure rare

A 19-year-old student was taken ill on a working summer vacation in Scandinavia. Over the course of 2 weeks, she became increasingly unwell, tired and short of breath. She rapidly became more short of breath and finally collapsed. In hospital, she was found to have an abnormal mitral valve. She underwent heart surgery, where a clot the size of a table tennis ball was found on the valve, and removed. She made a full recovery. She was subsequently found to be aPL positive.

Comment
There are two areas of the heart which can be affected in Hughes syndrome – the heart valves, and the heart's own coronary arteries.

One of the stranger aspects of APS in sicker, usually untreated patients is the development of heart valve lesions. In extreme cases, lumps of thrombosis (clot) develop on the valves, especially the mitral and aortic valves.

These can impair normal blood flow, and, more seriously, can dislodge and fly off to affect other organs.

This valve involvement is one of the many features which separates APS from other clotting disorders. Milder cases usually go undetected but are sometimes picked up as heart murmur on stethoscope examination of the chest. The diagnosis is more precisely confirmed by echocardiography – a painless and quick chest examination.

The majority of patients with mild disease require little therapy. Rarely, however, the development of valve thrombosis and damage can be dramatic, as in this patient.

Take Home Message
One of the causes of breathlessness in Hughes syndrome is heart valve disease. A simple echocardiograph is an important investigation.

CASE 26
The Blood

Easy Bruising ......

- Low platelet counts
- Bruising
- May require steroid treatment

A 33-year-old teacher had previously had two episodes of leg thrombosis and investigations had shown a positive aPL. He was treated at first with warfarin but subsequently with long-term low-dose aspirin (75 mg daily). Following a school cricket match, he noticed more-than-expected bruising on his legs. He then complained of excessive gum bleeding. Investigations showed a platelet count of 4,000 (normal: 150,000). He was treated for a period of 3 months with steroids (prednisolone) and the platelet count returned to normal. There has been no subsequent episode of low platelets.

Comment
Oddly enough there seem to be a group of aPL-positive individuals whose sole medical problem is with low platelet counts. Whether these patients have a different mechanism or different form of the disease is unclear at present.

The fact that individuals with aPL can both clot or (occasionally) bleed is hard to comprehend. The tendency for platelet numbers to fall (patients with Hughes syndrome often run a "borderline" platelet count between 100,000 and 120,000, for example) is unique to APS amongst the clotting disorders. It has led to a number of researchers suggesting that one of the mechanisms by which patients with APS spontaneously thrombose is due to an effect of the antibodies on the delicate platelet membrane.

Take Home Message
A very low platelet count leads to a risk of bruising and of bleeding and demands treatment with steroids or other medication – especially for the patient with underlying clotting problems which may require warfarin or heparin treatment.

CASE 27
The Adrenal Glands

Addison's Disease: 200 Years On?

- Clotting in adrenals
- Addison's disease
- A medical emergency

The adrenal glands are important in maintaining a variety of means of protection against stress. When the adrenal glands "fail," the common symptoms are of lethargy, fluid problems, and finally, coma.

In 1987, a young man taught us –dramatically – that the adrenals could be involved in the APS.

A 24-year-old male student was referred for advice regarding treatment. He had been diagnosed in Indonesia with APS, having suffered recurrent thrombosis, with positive aPL tests in Jakarta. Almost immediately on arrival in London, he developed a further thrombosis and was admitted to hospital. He was ill and drowsy and within 24 hours became unconscious.

The diagnosis was made by a very bright junior doctor on our team who suggested that the loss of consciousness was due to chemical (electrolyte) imbalance, possibly due to failure of the adrenal gland. The patient was treated successfully and subsequent investigation showed that both adrenal glands had failed, almost certainly due to clotting in the adrenal blood vessels.

This particular, dramatic, case stimulated a lot of interest in medical circles. Dr Ron Asherson, a senior clinical fellow who had joined my unit, collected, in seemingly no time at all, some 40 cases following our ward round discussions of this case. It so happened that a meeting on Addison's disease was being held at Guy's Hospital in London to commemorate the 200th anniversary of the birth of Thomas Addison (a Guy's doctor).

The causes of Addison's disease are varied (in the old days, tuberculosis was a major cause), but as usual, the commonest cause is "unknown." We were invited as a "late entry" to the Guy's meeting to present our data on APS as a cause (possibly an important cause) of Addison's disease.

Take Home Message
Some patients with Hughes syndrome develop very severe medical problems. Failure of the vital adrenal glands can be one cause – a treatable cause.

CASE 28
The Digestive System

Tummy Pain ......

- "Abdominal angina"
- Pain 1 hour after meals
- Poor gut circulation

If the heart arteries clot, you get chest pain. If the stomach arteries clot, you get stomach pain.

The blood supply to the gut has also been found compromised in some patients with **APS**. "Abdominal angina" is a condition which is difficult to diagnose, but sometimes the symptoms are very suggestive – stomach pain coming on some time after a meal.

A 62-year-old woman complained of increasingly severe stomach pains over a 2-year period. Barium meal and endoscopic examination of the esophagus, stomach and duodenum showed no abnormality. Over time, it became clear that the pain followed a meal by a clear interval of about 1 hour – a symptom sometimes suggestive of "ischemia" (i.e. not enough blood supply for the work of digestion). An X-ray investigation of the blood vessels (angiogram) showed an area of narrowing of a critical part of the major bowel artery. She was also noted clinically to have "livedo reticularis" of the skin and found to be aPL positive. She was treated surgically to remove the obstruction in the artery, and has since been on anticoagulants. The abdominal pain has gone.

Comment
We have now reported on a sizeable number of patients with Hughes syndrome with "abdominal angina." The characteristic appearance on X-ray angiography is of a localized narrowing in one of the main arteries supplying the gut. Some patients require surgery for this condition, but, as in this case, in some patients, improvement when blood-thinning medicine is started is striking.

Take Home Message
Abdominal pain an hour or so after a big meal can be due to an impaired blood supply to the intestines. Gastroenterologists are now seeing and treating Hughes syndrome.

CASE 29
The Reproductive System

Impotence ......

- Impotence – due to poor circulation
- Possibly under-reported

One feature of peripheral arterial disease which is recognized in other vascular diseases, but, to my knowledge, not yet described in Hughes syndrome, is impotence.

A 60-year-old male was referred to our APS clinic with previous thrombosis, skin "livedo reticularis," and worsening calf pains on walking. Until very recently, he had received no long-term treatment. Despite his many problems, the one development which concerned him most was of impotence – a problem which only came to light late on during the consultation. Significantly, this symptom was helped by the introduction of the drug sildenafil ("Viagra").

Comment
Impotence can be a problem in any disease which affects the circulation.

Artery disease is one of the major afflictions of Western society. Diet, cholesterol, smoking, lifestyle and genetics have all come under scrutiny. Now we have a new clue – a link between clotting or sludging of blood and the "furring up" of arteries. More importantly, it is a clue leading to possible earlier diagnosis or treatment in this group of patients.

Take Home Message
Every organ is dependent on a good circulation. Impotence is possibly an under-recognized feature of Hughes syndrome.

CASE 30
The Limbs

Severe Leg Pain ......

* Artery clots in legs
* Acute medical emergency

An 18-year-old boy, previously fit, and having recently won admission to university, complained of severe left calf pain. He rapidly developed painful discoloration of the foot and subsequently required amputation of the toes. Subsequent investigation revealed very high levels of aPL. He was treated with anticoagulants and has remained well (on anticoagulants) for the past two decades. For the whole of this period of observation, his aPL levels have remained high.

Comment
The fact that patients with Hughes syndrome can and do develop arterial as well as vein thrombosis is of immense clinical importance. Any artery can be affected including the largest arteries such as the carotid (neck), aorta, arm and leg arteries. The onset can be gradual, and relatively free of symptoms or dramatic, as in the case of this patient.

Take Home Message
A clot in an artery is a major medical emergency. While cases such as this are rare, aPL testing is vital for future management.

CASE 31
Pain in the Foot ("Toelitis")

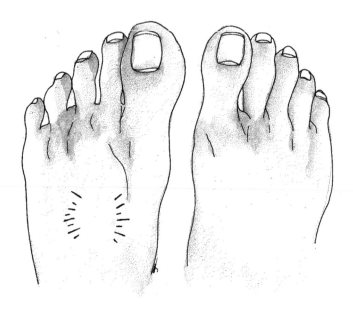

- Bone fracture...
- ...can happen without force
- Due to poor bone circulation

A 30-year-old man with Hughes syndrome (previous migraine and thrombosis in an arm vein, aPL positive) complained of persistent pain in the left foot. Putting weight on the foot was uncomfortable and walking was limited.

There had been no history of trauma, and any unusual sporting or leisure activity. On examination, there was tenderness over the bones of the left mid-foot region.

An X-ray, rather surprisingly, showed a fracture of the third metatarsal. Other bones were normal.

Comment

Is the fracture linked to APS? Probably yes. Dr. Shirish Sangle, one of my team, collected no less than 54 cases of spontaneous bone fracture in our patients with Hughes syndrome – during a surprisingly short period of time. Since then, a number of other cases of "spontaneous" fracture has been reported, including fractures in other bones including ribs and spinal fracture.

What is the mechanism? Although we are not certain, it seems likely that impaired blood supply (ischemia) to the bone underlies this problem.

Again, here is a medical discovery with important ramifications in yet another speciality – orthopedics. We have known for a long time that hip collapse (ischemic or avascular necrosis) can occur in patients with APS, presumably due to impaired circulation to the vulnerable "head" of the femur. Now we can add APS to the melting pot in the study of unexpected fractures.

Take Home Message
Spontaneous metatarsal fracture – "march fracture" – is a bizarre, yet not uncommon condition. The world of orthopedics is recognizing that in some cases of unexpected bone fracture, a clotting disorder such as Hughes syndrome can be responsible.

CASE 32
Ear, Nose and Throat

The Bells are Ringing

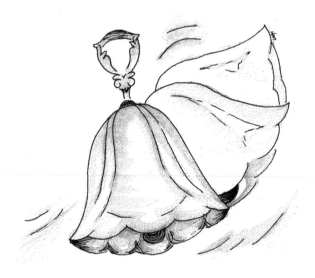

> • ENT symptoms...
> • ...can include "tinnitus"

A 46-year-old doctor's wife suffered an acute attack of vertigo, then attributed to middle ear infection or "Meniere's disease." However, her subsequent progress included a small stroke, recurrent balance problems and tinnitus (persistent ringing in the ears). She was finally diagnosed as Hughes syndrome and treated with warfarin. She responded well. Interestingly, the tinnitus all but disappeared with good warfarin control, returning whenever the INR fell below 2.5.

Comment
Tinnitus can be one of the most unpleasant and persistent symptoms known to man. Anecdotally, in my own practice, I am seeing an increasing number of patients with "ENT" and balance problems. Strikingly, in three of these patients, the tinnitus has improved

with warfarin treatment, suggesting that in these cases at least, "sticky blood" or sludging may well have contributed.

Take Home Message
One of my ENT colleagues in London is sending me more and more patients with balance problems, "middle ear" problems, "Meniere's disease" – due to "sticky blood."

The improvement in many of these symptoms when anticoagulant treatment is started is often dramatic (Figs. 32.1 32.2).

Hughes Syndrome Patients' Questionnaire Fig. 32.1

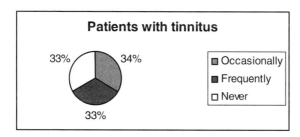

Fig. 32.2

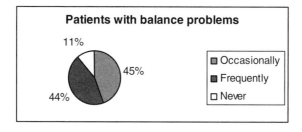

CASE 33
The Kidneys

Two Swollen Legs ......

> • Clots in kidney veins
> • ...can cause leg swelling
> • ...and, if untreated, kidney failure

A 34-year-old patient, at 35 weeks of pregnancy, developed severe weight gain, leg swelling and fluid retention. She was found to have high levels of protein in the urine. Investigations showed that she had thrombosis in the veins from both kidneys ("renal vein thrombosis"). The baby was delivered successfully, but the patient went on to develop severe kidney problems. She was anticardiolipin test positive on blood testing.

Comment
Renal vein thrombosis is a well-recognized acute medical problem. Again, the majority of cases have no known cause, but APS is now recognized as an important contributor in some cases.

The clinical picture is often dramatic – there is loin pain (the kidney becomes swollen) and the urine contains increasing amounts of leaked protein.

Sometimes, so much protein is lost that the body's metabolism is upset, leading to marked ankle swelling and fluid retention. The recognition of this rare complication of APS is vital as urgent treatment can save the kidney from permanent damage.

Take Home Message
Clotting in the kidney blood vessels can have dramatic consequences, including protein loss (as in this patient), raised blood pressure and, in untreated cases, kidney failure requiring dialysis.

CASE 34
"Multi-System Failure"
The computer has crashed.

(The "Catastrophic" APS)

- Widespread clotting
- Medical emergency
- "Triggering factor" often unknown

A 35-year-old woman, previously diagnosed as Hughes syndrome with leg vein thrombosis, previous spontaneous abortions, livedo reticularis, and a number of small strokes, had been successfully treated with warfarin (Coumadin) for 3 years and was doing very well. On Christmas Day, she was involved in a car crash, suffered head injuries and was admitted unconscious to a neurosurgical centre. Warfarin was stopped because of the danger of internal bleeding. After an initial improvement, she again started to become more drowsy and short of breath. A heart murmur was noted, and her liver function tests became abnormal. Her condition deteriorated rapidly, with lung and liver failure and worsening heart valve function. In collaboration with our unit, it was decided to restart anticoagulation. There was a clear and marked improvement. Two years later, she underwent corrective valve surgery. The patient remains well 9 years after the Christmas emergency, and on lifelong anticoagulants.

Comment
One of the most feared complications of Hughes syndrome is often known as "catastrophic" APS. Fortunately, it is extremely rare – but when it occurs it is an "all stops out" medical emergency.

The most commonly cited scenario is in an individual with aPL who appears to be well – often on no treatment – who suddenly starts to develop widespread clots. The clots involve any or all of the vital organs – the lungs, liver, the adrenals and the brain.

The patient becomes extremely ill and invariably requires intensive care treatment.

The triggering factor(s) for this "gear-change" is unknown; though in a number of patients an infection such as a virus, sore throat or chest infection seems to start the process. Another, rare, cause is the stopping of anticoagulant treatment in a known patient with aPL – almost certainly the case in the patient discussed here.

Because the catastrophic syndrome is so rare, there are few reports of successful treatment. Obviously, careful anticoagulation treatment is essential, as well as specialized intensive care management. Some studies have suggested that "blood-cleansing" (plasma exchange) might help by reducing the level of disease-producing antibodies. This makes good sense, but hard evidence for the success of this treatment is still lacking.

Take Home Message
Catastrophic APS, widespread organ thrombosis, requires the highest skills of the intensive care unit. Fortunately, it is a fairly rare event in Hughes syndrome.

Section 3
Pregnancy, Miscarriage, Infertility

CASE 35
Eleven Miscarriages

- Recurrent miscarriage
- Hughes syndrome a major cause
- Preventable!

A 39-year-old woman had suffered 11 spontaneous miscarriages. Following a clinical meeting on antiphospholipid syndrome (APS) in 1983, her physician in Scotland sent blood to us for antiphospholipid (aPL) testing and she was positive. She was treated with 75-mg aspirin daily plus subcutaneous daily heparin and completed a successful pregnancy (followed by a second 1 year later).

This patient – a woman whose courage and determination was finally rewarded –used to travel down to London for her check-ups on the overnight train – a 20 hour round trip!

Comment
A woman with recurrent pregnancy loss *must* be checked for Hughes syndrome, as this is an important and preventable cause.

One of the most important aspects of Hughes syndrome has been its impact on obstetrics. APS is now regarded as the *commonest, treatable* cause of recurrent miscarriage. The mechanisms for pregnancy loss are still being debated, though clearly thrombosis of placental blood vessels plays an important part. Almost from the start of pregnancy, the placenta vessels silt up, the fetus starved of oxygen and miscarriage follows.

The recognition of this important cause of miscarriage has had a profound impact. Pregnancy success rates have been turned around from a miserable 15% 20 years ago, to over 90% in most clinics now dealing with the problem.

While much of the success has come from careful use of aspirin and/or heparin, a significant contribution to this undoubted success story has come from the evolution of combined obstetric/medical clinics – especially in the prevention of the tragedy of late pregnancy loss.

Take Home Message
A "new" syndrome – only 25 years old – yet now recognized as the commonest treatable cause of recurrent pregnancy loss.

CASE 36
Late Pregnancy Tragedy ......

> • *Late* pregnancy loss...
> • ...is also seen in Hughes syndrome
> • Always check for aPL

Mrs. D.B., aged 28, had been doing well in her second pregnancy. Her first pregnancy had ended in miscarriage at 3 months. At around 7 months, things started to go wrong, with a rise in blood pressure and slight ankle swelling. Soon afterwards, a Doppler monitor showed that the fetus' blood supply was rapidly becoming impaired.

Emergency caesarean section was carried out, but the newborn infant was dead.

At that time the mother had not been tested for aPL, but subsequent testing showed her to be strongly positive.

A year later, under the care of the combined lupus pregnancy team at St. Thomas' hospital, on daily heparin injections and with regular Doppler monitoring, she gave birth to a healthy girl.

Comment
Early pregnancy loss is due to a variety of causes including uterine abnormalities and chromosome defects, as well as APS. By contrast, *late* pregnancy loss should always raise the suspicion of Hughes syndrome. Again, this case, as in so many like it, supports the argument for regular aPL testing in pregnancy. So little the cost. So great the gain.

Take Home Message
Late pregnancy loss – always test for aPL.

CASE 37
The Infertility Clinic

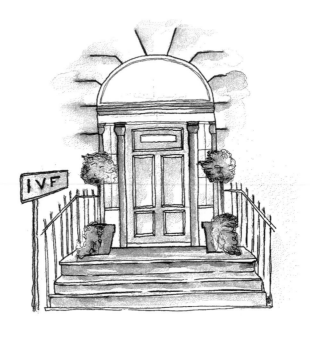

> • Recurrent *early* pregnancy loss...
> • ...can cause "infertility"
> • Aspirin/heparin may help

Mrs. J.R., aged 28, and her 30-year-old husband had tried three courses of in vitro fertilization (IVF) having failed to conceive. A fourth attempt, at a different clinic, was successful. Three years later following a deep vein thrombosis (DVT), she was found to be aPL positive.

Comment

Controversy seems to be the bedfellow of IVF. Firstly, current studies are divided as to whether the problem of infertility is common in aPL-positive individuals. Logic would suggest that it is, with recurrent early miscarriage and placental implantation problems being known associations. Likewise, there is disagreement on whether the addition of aspirin or heparin to the IVF regime produces more successful pregnancies.

As fate would have it, this patient's fourth IVF attempt was in a clinic in which heparin was added. We await more detailed and larger studies to answer the question as to whether there is a significant link between "sticky blood" and infertility.

Take Home Message
As well as miscarriage and late pregnancy loss, aPL may also result in repeated very early loss, failure of implantation and problems of infertility. While some cases of infertility are associated with aPL, it is clear that more studies in this area are needed.

Section 4
Causes and Effects

THE "TWO HIT" THEORY

Hughes syndrome is classed as an "autoimmune" disease – a condition in which proteins called "antibodies" are important players. Whether or not these antibodies *cause* the disease is debatable, but in the case of a number of diseases, the link is strong – for example, thyroid antibodies and thyroid disease or anti-Ro antibodies and congenital heart block in some offspring of patients with lupus.

So, similarly aPL (antiphospholipid) antibodies, conventionally measured by two tests, aCL (anticardiolipin antibodies) and LA (the confusingly termed lupus anticoagulant – *NOT* a test for lupus!) are strongly associated with thrombosis.

As with other autoimmune disease, there is clear evidence of a genetic tendency in Hughes syndrome, though this is not a strong one.

It is also clear that the tendency to clot is heightened by other well-known suspects, including smoking, dehydration, prolonged immobilization and the oral contraceptive.

Lastly, in others, there may be a "second hit" – an unexpected factor such as infection. Some examples are given here.

CASE 38
'The Pill and I......'

- "Second hits" may be needed
- One such risk is the contraceptive pill

A 17-year-old girl was started on the oral contraceptive pill. There were no known predisposing risk factors for thrombosis with the one possible exception – a history of previous occasional migraine attacks, present since the age of 13.

Within 2 weeks of starting the pill she collapsed. She was found to have major thrombosis in the leg veins with the spread of the clot to the pelvic veins and the lungs. She survived following a prolonged period of intensive care. She has high levels of aPL and has since been treated successfully with warfarin (Coumadin). Three years later, aPL levels remain high and warfarin treatment continues. She is now married and considering pregnancy.

Comment

The issues raised by this case concerns not only treatment but also the wider and important issue of prevention (should migraine sufferers be tested for aPL? – yes, in my opinion).

The oral contraceptive has long been associated with an increased tendency to thrombosis: it may well be that those with aPL antibodies are especially at risk. Again, a case could be made for aPL as a screening health check.

Take Home Message

The oral contraceptive pill, especially the high estrogen pill, increases the risk of thrombosis. Clearly, women with positive aPL are particularly vulnerable.

CASE 39
A Bad Back ......

> • Pre-existing poor circulation...
> • ...can be worsened by sticky blood

A 61-year-old lady with a long history of back troubles had had her ups and downs with treatment. Recently, however, things had deteriorated, with increasing difficulty in walking. She could now only manage 100 yards or so before having to stop because of leg pains.

She was investigated and diagnosed as having a condition called "spinal stenosis" – wear and tear in the back resulting in the bottom end of the spine being narrowed and affecting the nerve supply to the legs.

By coincidence, she was also being investigated for heart flutters – "atrial fibrillation." Amongst the positive investigations was a persistently strongly positive aPL test. It was decided to treat her with warfarin anticoagulation. Within a matter of days, the walking improved – distances of a quarter of a mile and more were no problem.

Comment
Coincidence? Or was this patient teaching us something? Often in medicine, there is more than one diagnosis, and sometimes the problems of each are additive. In this patient, it is certainly possible that the cutting off of blood supply to the nerves in legs due to the lumbar disc problem was critical to an already compromised oxygen supply resulting from "sticky blood."

Take Home Message
"Sticky blood" almost certainly worsened the leg pains by adding to the circulation problems.

The next case highlights this "two hit" phenomenon even more strikingly.

CASE 40
"A Miracle"......

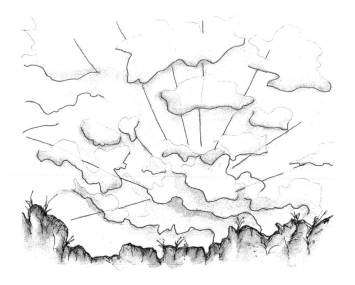

- Impaired circulation affecting spinal cord
- Dramatic improvement in treatment

Mrs. C.L., a 36-year-old housewife, had become progressively paralyzed in both legs, and wheelchair bound. She had developed incontinence of urine, and leg spasms which were so severe that on one occasion she was thrown from her wheelchair, breaking a bone.

She was thought to have multiple sclerosis particularly targeting the spinal cord.

Investigations carried out at the neurology hospital in Queen Square, London, however, turned up a surprise – a small blood vessel abnormality in the spinal cord – a so-called arteriovenous shunt. The mystery remained, however, as the small abnormality was not consistent with the degree of disability.

During this period of investigation, she developed a leg clot – a small deep vein thrombosis (DVT), and was started on warfarin. The result was dramatic – within days the spasms had lessened, and within weeks she was walking.

She is now perfectly fit (on lifelong warfarin) and able to walk, run and even dance. She became an active member of the Hughes Syndrome Foundation charity.

Comment

Here, surely is a clear cut example of the interaction of two risk factors contributing together to severely compromise the blood supply of the spinal cord.

Take Home Message

Even the most dramatic symptoms such as paralysis can respond to the right treatment!

CASE 41
Climbing the Andes ......

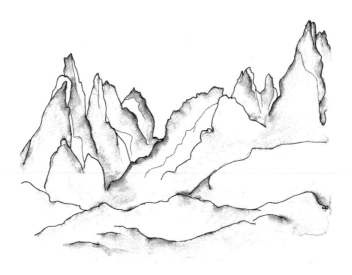

- aPL positive – previously healthy
- Clotting at high altitude

A 22-year-old medical student, whilst on a climbing expedition high in the Andes, collapsed, became unconscious, and recovered only after being given emergency treatment and hospital management at lower altitude. Subsequent investigations showed that he had developed a brain thrombosis in one of the veins of the brain – so-called saggital sinus thrombosis. He was aPL positive.

Comment
This case is interesting in possibly supporting the "two-hit" hypothesis in Hughes syndrome – the underlying problems ("sticky blood") and the precipitating factor – in this case possibly high altitude and its associated metabolic changes.

While vein thrombosis can and does occasionally affect the brain, the main concern with this organ, and, indeed, for all patients with Hughes syndrome, is the risk of arterial clots or strokes. It is this threat which makes diagnosis and screening for

APS so important, and decisions concerning duration and intensity of treatment so critical.

In a perverse way, the brain can be viewed as a simple organ. If angered or insulted, it is capable of reacting in fairly limited, well-defined ways.

Just as the car engine starved of fuel either stutters or stops, so the brain, is given limited blood (and hence oxygen) supply, complains in ways well recognized by the neurologist. The most dramatic and serious, of course, is a stroke, with weakness down one side of the body and possibly with effects of speech. More localized ischemia (poor circulation) can lead to a wide variety of features including seizures, migraine, visual disturbance and spinal cord problems.

Some patients present with less "dramatic" symptoms – such as memory loss, loss of sensation (sometimes leading to a mistaken diagnosis of "MS") and movement disorders (including chorea- "St Vitus Dance").

Take Home Message
Although the threat of development of a stroke is the biggest fear, one wonders how many individuals with more subtle forms of brain involvement are either being misdiagnosed or not being diagnosed at all.

The next case, while not offering proof, suggests that less dramatic influences might also contribute in some cases.

CASE 42
Fear of Flying ......

- Flying normally safe
- Untreated aPL-positive individuals at greater risk!

In retrospect, Mrs. G.H. had had features suggestive of Hughes syndrome for many years: one previous vein thrombosis ("DVT") previous migraine headaches and a long history of aches and pains. Clinical examination was revealing. She had a bone dry Schirmer's test (a simple blotting paper test to determine tear secretion – "dry eyes" are a feature of Sjögren syndrome). She also had florid livedo reticularis – "corned beef skin" – a blotchy appearance of the skin suggesting poor circulation.

Her "aviation history" was dramatic. Every time she flew on a journey of over a couple of hours, she became ill – nauseated, short of breath, achy for 2–3 days. She attributed the symptoms to stress, though flying did not worry her.

When she was finally diagnosed with Hughes syndrome, and started on aspirin, the post-flight illness became less severe. Finally, on the advice of her physician, she tried a subcutaneous heparin injection before a long haul flight. The effect was dramatic. No more "long haul illness".

Comment
This story is typical of many of our patients. The combination of Sjögren syndrome (aches and pains, fatigue, allergies, dry eyes and mouth) and Hughes syndrome (headache, shortness of breath, memory loss, balance disturbance) is a daunting one – difficult to diagnose and certainly difficult to live with.

The patient genuinely improved with anticoagulation. She was a frequent flyer – her husband worked in aviation, and commented that despite the outstanding commitment of aviation safety, cost cutting did sometimes lead to cut corners – for example, in the quality of aeration of cabin air. Imperceptible in most, it is just conceivable that it would make a difference in someone with compromised oxygen supply through circulation.

(One of my patients with Hughes syndrome, an eminent Professor of Medicine, noticed that on holiday with her husband in the Swiss Alps, she was predictably prone to increasing headaches with every thousand meters of altitude).

Take Home Message
Although flying is safe for most people (including the majority with various illnesses), there is clearly a need for a study of the effects in treated versus non-treated patients with Hughes syndrome.

CASE 43
The Lambeth Walk

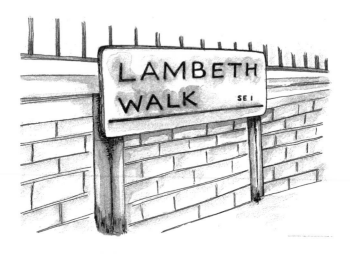

- Calf pain on walking ("claudication")...
- ...a common medical problem...
- ...can be due to Hughes syndrome
- Check the family history

Just behind St. Thomas' Hospital lies Lambeth walk, made famous by the cockney tune "Doing the Lambeth walk." Although things are changing rapidly, Lambeth has traditionally been a relatively poor working class area of London. The next case, that of a 60-year-old man from Lambeth, with intermittent leg pain and minor strokes, seemed commonplace enough – but with some surprises.

A 60-year-old man came to out-patients accompanied by his daughter. He had complained of calf pains on walking any distance and only relieved by resting (often known medically as "intermittent claudication"). He had also suffered a number of "TIAs" (transient ischemic attacks or mini-strokes). His blood pressure was normal. He was a non-smoker. However, blood tests had turned up a high level of aPL on two previous clinic visits, as well as multiple "UBOs" (unidentified bright objects) – small oxygen-starved areas – on brain magnetic resonance imaging (MRI). Leg Doppler showed impaired

*leg artery circulation. In the absence of other risk factors, a diagnosis
of probable APS was made and he was started on warfarin.*

Doctor: "Anybody else in your family with anything similar?"
Patient: "No, doc."
Daughter: "Come on, dad, you know there is ….."

*And, bit by bit, a striking family history unraveled. Dad was one
of 14 siblings. Of these, four had had thromboses, seven migraines,
two were diagnosed as multiple sclerosis and one had rheumatoid
arthritis. He had three daughters, one of whom had lupus and a
second – the daughter who accompanied dad – who was my patient
(primary APS with recurrent previous miscarriage) – hence the diagnosis being reached.*

Comment

Studies of the genetics of a disease are normally helped by studies
of large families with that condition. One geneticist told me that
the study of a disease in a family of 14 or more siblings, half of
whom had that condition, would be sufficient to almost certainly
identify the gene causing that disease.

Take Home Message

*The family history is important. Conditions as diverse as multiple
sclerosis, rheumatoid arthritis, migraine and thrombosis may be
connected. They certainly are in Hughes syndrome.*

CASE 44
"The Tests are Negative!"

- Blood tests valuable, but not infallible
- Ongoing research for newer, sensitive tests

Mrs. S.A, a 46-year-old housewife and previous medical receptionist, had developed symptoms of fatigue, mental "fuzziness," slight balance disorder. She had also developed frequent headaches – something she had not suffered for over 30 years. She also complained of (mild) aches and pains.

Investigations, including a brain MRI, were negative. No firm diagnosis was reached, though she received short periods of treatment of depression, and of fibromyalgia.

Because her sister had lupus and attended our lupus clinic, Mrs. S.A. finally made it to the same clinic.

The past history was interesting. After investigations for infertility, she finally became pregnant but suffered two miscarriages and, tragically, one late fetal death. Following this, she developed a probable DVT though this was not proven. The family history included, as well as the sister with lupus, a sister with under-active thyroid, and an aunt with thyroid problems.

Examination revealed two important findings – the now familiar pairing of dry eyes (bone-dry "Schirmer's" blotting paper test), and fairly marked skin livedo reticularis (blotchy mottling).

All tests for autoimmune disease (apart from a positive anti-nuclear antibody "ANA") were negative. All clotting tests, including a full aPL antibody screen, were also negative.

Comment

What is the diagnosis? How should she be managed? The answer in this case seemed to be easy – apart from the problem of the negative tests. This patient had a strong family history of autoimmune disease, a past history of late pregnancy loss, two early miscarriages, and a possible DVT. In addition, she had two important physical signs – skin livedo reticularis and the dry eye finding, suggesting Sjögren syndrome.

Her case ended in "success." Low-dose aspirin immediately improved the headaches and "brain fogginess." She was also started on quinine – low-dose Plaquenil – with almost total improvement in the fatigue.

Take Home Message

We have introduced the term "sero-negative APS" – that is, the clinical features fit but the serum tests do not.

There are three possible reasons for negative tests in this situation. Firstly, the diagnosis is wrong, which is unlikely in this case. Secondly, previously positive tests might have become negative over the years – something we occasionally do see. Thirdly, possibly we are not sophisticated enough in our tests. It may be that bright young research doctors in the future will devise new, more specific tests for this family of autoimmune diseases.

There can be no better stimulus for such research than the success story provided by this patient – who might just have ended up with a wrong label of "depression" or "fibromyalgia."

Section 5
Aspects of Treatment

CASE 45
"My Sister has Hughes Syndrome"

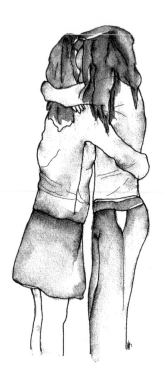

- Family history is important
- Even when the case is not "classical"

An 18-year-old girl was referred by her general practitioner (GP), complaining of unexplained fatigue and frequent headaches. The symptoms appeared to have started 2 years earlier following a bout of glandular fever.

She had been reluctant to see her GP, attributing the symptoms to stress in her office job, but had finally been persuaded by her sister, aged 25, a patient with known Hughes syndrome.

The GP acceded to her requests and detailed tests showed positive aPL (antiphospholipid) tests and ANA (anti-nuclear antibodies)

– further evidence of an autoimmune tendency. She also had positive thyroid antibody tests. DNA antibody testing for lupus was negative. Later, tests included a normal brain scan.

She was treated with "baby" aspirin and later with low-dose Plaquenil – a quinine derivative – with complete disappearance of the symptoms.

Comment

This patient underlines the importance of tests (and of taking a full family history). They show a strong background of autoimmune problems. The negative DNA antibody test is strongly against lupus but other tests are important. The thyroid antibodies point to increased risk of thyroid problems (especially an underactive thyroid); the ANA is common in milder lupus variants such as Sjögren syndrome (dry mouth, dry eyes, aches and pains, fatigue and allergies) while the positive aPL led to the successful introduction of Aspirin. Plaquenil (a quinine medicine which, like aspirin, is derived from the bark of a tree) is very useful for treating fatigue in autoimmune conditions such as Sjögren syndrome and lupus.

This case also highlights the importance of "listening to the patient." This patient's rather non-specific symptoms of fatigue and headache could so easily have been dismissed.

Take Home Message

A family history of Hughes syndrome, thyroid or lupus should always be taken seriously.

CASE 46
Trial and Error

- If the suspicion is strong…
- …treatment is always worth trying

Over the years, I have observed that if a patient with Hughes syndrome develops a thrombosis, and starts anticoagulation, there is often an immediate and striking improvement in some of the "general" features of the syndrome, notably the headaches and brain "fuzziness."

While aspirin is a safe and available treatment, warfarin carries more dangers and has far wider implications. Clearly, the decision to try warfarin in a patient without prior thrombosis is almost impossibly difficult. Heparin, however, might be different.

Miss D.L., aged 34, was diagnosed with Hughes syndrome. She had had childhood and teenage migraine – a problem which had recurred in her late 20s. There was also a past history of chorea, of visual disturbance and of balance problems. There was florid livedo reticularis. She had strongly positive aPL tests. Brain magnetic resonance imaging (MRI) was normal. Her main complaint, however, was of memory loss: she found it difficult to remember words and often came out with the totally wrong word for a particular object. Her partner and she were concerned about possible Alzheimer's.

She had been on junior aspirin (75 mg daily) for some years, but it seemed to have little impact on her symptoms.

Around this time, we had a young doctor from St. Thomas' psychiatric department attending our clinic, with a research project including psychometry in our patients. Full psychometric analysis is a specialized and time-consuming process and includes many parameters, one of which is word finding.

Miss D.L. had a normal I.Q., but her word finding ability was down to the 14th percentile…. She truly could not string words together.

For a 3-week trial period, we changed the aspirin to heparin (low-molecular-weight heparin subcutaneously self-administered daily – a treatment carried out for up to 9 months by some of our pregnant patients with Hughes syndrome).

She was tested at the end of 3 weeks. The same word finding test was repeated: This time the result was over 90! A staggering outcome. Clinically, not only was there a huge improvement in memory but also the headaches virtually disappeared.

The patient has since converted to warfarin and remains well.

Comment

Faced with a patient with severe APS-related problems (such as increasingly severe hemiplegic migraine, for example), aspirin, the first choice of medicine, is often less than fully effective.

As a way of trying treatment less extreme than warfarin, we have devised, and published, a short-term "heparin trial" – usually 3 weeks of low-molecular-weight heparin. While the results are sometimes inconclusive, in others, such as Miss D.L., they clearly point us in the right direction. Perhaps in future, use of newer more sensitive brain-scanning techniques will give more exact help.

Take Home Message

It may be that few cases are as dramatic as this. Nevertheless, proper psychometric testing as in this patient possibly underlies the clinical impression of the frequency and importance of memory loss in patients with Hughes syndrome.

CASE 47
"I Saved the Country £73,000"

- Medicine control is critical
- Self-testing of warfarin control ("INR") useful...
- ...especially in Hughes syndrome

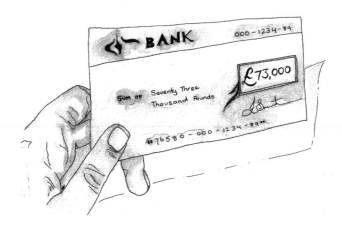

A 36-year-old woman complained of headaches, speech disturbance, visual impairment, lethargy and episodes of loss of consciousness lasting up to 10 minutes. A brain scan showed numerous small, well-defined white matter lesions. Blood tests revealed strongly positive anticardiolipin antibody (aCL). Her history included three early mis-carriages 14 years earlier, two possible deep vein thrombosis (DVTs), and an unproved pulmonary embolism 3 years previously. A diagnosis of Hughes syndrome (APS) was made and treated with warfarin, with immediate improvement in symptoms. Anticoagulation control was difficult, however, with the international normalized ratio (INR) fluctuating significantly.

She was certain that the symptoms (including the loss of con-sciousness) returned when the INR fell below a critical 2.8. With half-day round trip to her anticoagulant clinic, and erratic INR control, she suffered seven hospital admissions in 1999 for various thrombosis-related events: She campaigned for, and received, an INR self-testing machine. By her own admission, her life has changed. Any return headaches or other neurological feature is met with an immediate INR test and, when necessary, fine-tuning of warfarin. From seven hospital admission in 1999, there were none in 2000.

Confidence to travel abroad has returned, and the fear of further transient ischemic attack or strokes receded.

Comment

In this case, there are a number of lessons. Recurrent miscarriage in a patient with APS may still harbor clotting problems years later. Neurological features, notably headaches (or memory loss), are important. APS is an important cause of stroke. Improvement with anticoagulation can be striking. Careful INR control with warfarin is critical – indeed, many patients with brain symptoms require an INR of 3 or even more. Self-testing of INR, as in the case of self-testing diabetes, could have important medical as well as health economic benefits, especially in such a prothrombotic disorder.

During the year 1999, she had seven admissions to hospital for thrombosis. Home self-testing with an INR self-testing machine was suggested, but she could ill afford the £300 needed. A local newspaper took up her case and the money was found. She rapidly learned to control her own warfarin "fine-tuning," and the following year, there were no further thrombosis.

Cost to the country of one machine: £300. Cost to the country of her seven hospital admissions: £73,000!

In the UK at least, self-testing of INR is the exception rather than the rule. And yet in those patients with Hughes syndrome, and erratic INRs, the move to self-testing has been a blessing. As one business woman said "It has set me free. I can go to all corners of the world without worrying. The return of any headache or mental 'fogginess' simply triggers a finger prick INR check and fine adjustment of the dose."

For me, this is the future of warfarin control – in the same way that young diabetics on insulin now take charge of their own lives.

Take Home Message

Diabetics are quite capable of managing their own sugar and insulin control. Why should not patients with Hughes syndrome who are on warfarin similarly self-check?

CASE 48
What Happened Next?

- Choice of aspirin vs heparin vs warfarin not always easy
- Sometimes "trial and error" the only way

A 29-year-old woman from Athens was referred for a second opinion regarding treatment of Hughes syndrome. She had a past history of headaches from the age of 9, of Raynaud's (cold hands and feet), and from the age of 16, muscle and joint aches and pains. Her overriding complaint was fatigue. The family history included a sister with an underactive thyroid, and her father with stroke. Investigations included positive aCL and negative tests for lupus.

She had been started on aspirin with some improvement, the headaches being less frequent. However, fatigue remained a major symptom.

A 3-week course of heparin was tried. This resulted in clear-out improvement. However, as she had never suffered a thrombosis, warfarin was thought inappropriate. She returned to Athens on aspirin.

What happened next?

Back in Athens, she persuaded her physician, a family friend, to start her on warfarin, with careful INR monitoring.

The result was striking. Not only did the headaches stop but the fatigue and muscle aches also vanished. Some 9 months into this treatment, she required dental treatment. Warfarin was stopped for a week – with immediate return of the headaches, fatigue and muscle aches.

Comment

The doubter could agree that symptoms such as headache, fatigue and muscle aches might well respond to placebo treatment and there is no doubt that a daily self-injection (heparin) could have an important placebo effect – "that something is being done."

However, our experience over the past 20 years has included far too many stories similar to our Greek patient to be due to chance.

One of the interesting lessons this patient (and many others) teaches us is that improving blood flow in Hughes syndrome not only helps headaches and memory loss but also fatigue, and – inexplicably, perhaps aches and pains.

Take Home Message

Some (possibly many) patients with Hughes syndrome respond better to warfarin than to aspirin or heparin. We desperately need tests which could help to pre-identify such patients.

CASE 49
"Your Condition Doesn't Exist"

- Hughes syndrome is…
- …a "new" disease (25 years old)
- …both
- Education is essential…
- …for both doctors and for patients

Diseases such as Hughes syndrome, Sjögren syndrome and mild lupus (what I call "The Big Three"*) are often difficult to diagnose and often lead to skepticism.

A 58-year-old woman complained of tiredness, mild muscle aches and memory problems. She had mild Reynaud's syndrome for many years and had reached the menopause 10 years previously. Although depression had been suggested, both she and her family were certain this was not the diagnosis.

Sadly, she had visited a number of doctors, one of whom looking up from his desktop told her "your condition doesn't exist."

Some 2 years later, following a worsening of symptoms she was found to have high (extraordinarily high) aCL levels and responded strikingly to low-dose aspirin.

Comment
Firstly, the diagnosis can be elusive. Patients sometimes complain that their doctors do not listen or believe them, but "your disease doesn't exist" was a new one on me.

Secondly, despite the very high levels of antibodies, this patient responded to aspirin alone. Whether this will remain sufficient treatment in the future remains to be seen.

Take Home Message
Having a "new" disease can be double trouble. Although Hughes syndrome is only 25 years old, it has still not reached many textbooks.

CASE 50
"I've Got My Life Back!"

> • Sometimes 'small' medicines – such as quinine and aspirin...
> • ...can profoundly improve life quality
> • ...especially in Sjögren's and Hughes syndromes

Often in medicine there is more than one condition causing symptoms – either coincidentally or by known association. One common "pairing" is of Hughes syndrome with Sjögren's syndrome (dry eyes, dry mouth, aches and pains and fatigue). Attention to the detail of both conditions can have a huge clinical impact.

A 57-year-old solicitor was a "high achiever," having become a partner in one of London's most prestigious law firms. She had had a long history of migraines, but these had not halted her career progress. For the past 2 years, however, she had suffered aches and pains ("rheumatism"), stiffness in the joints and muscles, severe fatigue and an increase in the frequency of her headaches. To add to her woes, she had developed definite memory lapses. She was pessimistic about holding onto her job and seriously planning to take early retirement.

Examination revealed one important clue – a bone dry tear test (a blotting paper hooked over the lower eyelid – normally soaking – proved completely dry after 5 minutes). Blood tests confirmed the presence of Sjögren's syndrome (positive antibody tests for ANA and "Ro") – and a very strongly positive aCL test.

She was started on low-dose aspirin, and, for the aches and pains and fatigue of Sjögren's, on quinine ("Plaquenil" 1 tablet a day).

Improvement was significant. Both the Hughes syndrome features (headache and memory loss) and the Sjögren's symptoms – rheumatism, fatigue improved strikingly.

Such was the improvement at 6 months that the solicitor was back fully at work and confident. In her words "I've got my life back!"

Comment
Aches and pains are common complaints in patients with Hughes syndrome. In many patients, they are more probably due to Sjögren's syndrome (a form of mild lupus) rather than to sticky blood. Plaquenil, a medicine derived from quinine, is a very useful treatment – safe, mild and effective.

Take Home Message

Medicine does not have to be dramatic, complex or expensive to achieve results. In this patient, two simple pills, aspirin and Plaquenil (both extracted from trees – the willow and the cinchona) had a profound effect on this patient's life.

Section 6
Conclusions: Random Thoughts

In the 25 years since our description of the antiphospholipid syndrome (Hughes syndrome/APS), the ramifications have rippled into all corners of medicine. In the field of obstetrics, it has had a profound effect, with one in five of all women with recurrent miscarriage having this potentially treatable condition.

The figure "1 in 5" keeps coming up in published clinical studies of APS – 1 in 5 of all deep vein thromboses (DVTs) cases, 1 in 5 cases of young strokes (under the age of 45) and 1 in 5 cases of "idiopathic" teenage epilepsy. In other conditions, we know that Hughes syndrome can be one of the causes, but we do not know exactly how important a cause. Such conditions include migraine, memory loss and Alzheimer's, leg ulcers, young heart attacks, Meniere's disease.

The financial implications of the syndrome are huge – not to mention the clinical applications. What would the savings be of routine antiphospholipid (aPL) testing before surgery (e.g. post-operative DVT is still a major problem following hip and knee replacement surgery), in the case of chronic leg ulcers, or in the investigation of memory loss?

And in the world of research, there are already major ongoing studies of newer treatment, the role of aPL in arterial disease in general and the effects of aPL on brain, blood vessels and placenta – to name but three.

As far as treatment is concerned, the reader may well have been disappointed in the seemingly narrow range of options – aspirin (a very "mundane" drug), heparin (an injection) or warfarin ("rat poison"). However, there are strong grounds for optimism. Firstly, the more judicious use of currently available treatments (e.g. self-testing in some patients on warfarin) has already helped many hundreds of patients. Secondly, new treatments are coming over the horizon – for example, selective immunosuppressive drugs to knock out the antibody-producing cells, new tablet-form heparin substitutes. Some of the newer drugs may fall by the wayside. But such is the frequency and importance of Hughes syndrome, there is now major (and international) collaboration in newer ways of treating the condition.

The quote at the beginning of this volume talks of APS as a "new" disease. There is a downside to any "new" disease. Doctors will need to learn of its existence. To learn of its implications and of its presence in almost all corners of medicine. For those of us working in this field, it is an important part of our work to contribute towards that learning.

I hope that this short volume with its 50 illustrative cases will help both doctors and patients alike.

A new syndrome?

O*ver the past 11 years at the Hammersmith Hospital, I have seen a number of patients who appear to me to have a distinct syndrome or a set of features. These have been referred to in previous Hammersmith meetings and publications, but this lecture gives me the opportunity to discuss the constellation of features in detail, and, to suggest certain pathogenic mechanisms.*

Although many of these patients fall under the general heading of lupus, or lupus-like disease, I believe that the group is sufficiently homogeneous, and in some ways (such as the frequently negative

Table: A common syndrome
Multiple thromboses
Multiple abortions
Cerebral disease
Livedo reticularis
Thrombocytopenia
Serological features
ANA often negative
Anticardiolipin antibodies common

ANA. serology) sufficiently different from systemic lupus erythematosus (SLE) to warrant separate consideration.

The manifestations of this syndrome are thromboses (often multiple) and, frequently, spontaneous abortions (often multiple), neurological disease, thrombocytopenia (low platelets) and livedo reticularis. The livedo reticularis is often most florid on the knees. This may or may not be associated with mild-to-moderate Raynaud's phenomenon.

These patients' blood pressures often fluctuate, apparently correlating with the severity of the livedo, suggesting a possible renovascular aetiology. However, this group of patients rarely has primary renal disease.

---

[1] *Taken from the original 1983 description.*
[2] *With kind permission of Blackwell Publishing. Taken from the 1983 Prosser White oration. Published in Clinical & Experimental, Dermatology 1984, 9, 535–544.*

The cerebral features are prominent, and of three varieties:

Headaches – *often migrainous and intractable.*
Epilepsy (or abnormal EEGs) – *often going back to early teenage. Fortunately, severe or difficult-to-control epilepsy is infrequent. Some patients have chorea.*
Cerebrovascular accidents – *sometimes transient and seemingly attribute to migraine, but frequently progressive. It is this aspect of the syndrome which I believe to be particularly significant and to which I shall return in this paper. The patients may develop transient cerebral ischemia attacks or visual defects, or, more significantly, progressive cerebral ischemia.*

Two other features of the syndrome are a tendency to multiple spontaneous abortions and peripheral thrombosis, often with multiple leg and arm vein thrombosis. We have also seen Budd-Chiari syndrome and renal vein thrombosis in some of these patients.

To my mind, the most striking, and often most serious feature of the disease is the tendency to thrombosis, particularly cerebral thrombosis. So prominent has this feature been that we have some patients in their 40s and 50s who had been diagnosed as primary cerebrovascular disease - or when - the labile hypertension has been observed - as hypertensive cerebrovascular disease.

The finding that many of these patients have high titres of circulating anticardiolipin antibodies leads us to believe that a new line of investigation may be possible in such patients.

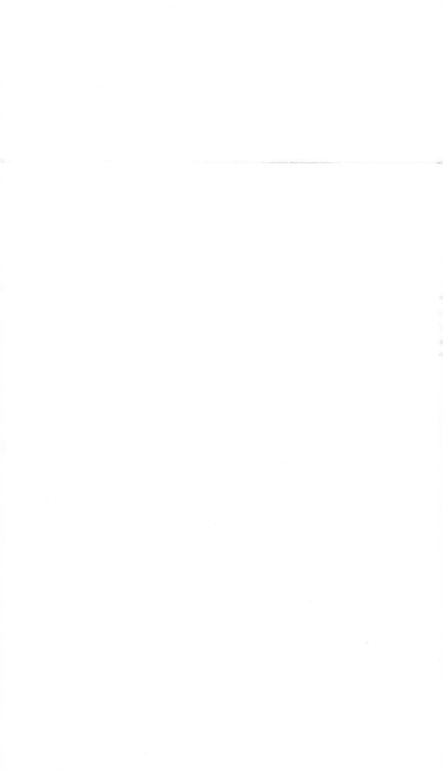

Printed in the United States of America